# COMPLETE GUIDE TO DENTAL IMPLANT SURGERY

Comprehensive Manual To Advanced Techniques, Recovery, and Best Practices for Optimal Oral Health

## DR. BRUNO HORAN

Copyright © 2023 by Dr. Bruno Horan

All rights reserved. Except for brief quotations embodied in critical reviews and certain other noncommercial uses permitted by copyright law, no part of this publication may be reproduced, distributed, or transmitted in any form or by any means, Including photocopying, recording, or other electronic or mechanical methods, without the prior written permission of the publisher.

## Disclaimer:

The information provided in this book, is intended for general informational purposes only and should not be considered as professional advice.

The author has made every effort to ensure the accuracy of the information presented. However, readers are advised to consult with a qualified healthcare professional before attempting any herbal remedies or making significant changes to their wellness routine. Individual health conditions vary, and what may be suitable for one person may not be appropriate for another.

It is important to note that the author is not in any endorsement deal, partnership, or affiliation with any organization, brand, or company mentioned in this book. Any references to specific products or services are based on the author's personal experience or general knowledge and do not imply an endorsement or promotion of those products or services

# Contents

CHAPTER ONE ................................................... 19

  PROCEDURES FOR DIAGNOSIS AND TREATMENT PLANNING .................................................... 19

    First Appointment And Evaluation Of The Patient 19

    Utilization Of Diagnostic Imaging (CT And X-Rays) ........................................................................... 20

    Software And Tools For Digital Planning ............. 21

    Formulating A Personalized Therapy Program ..... 22

    Estimating Costs And Taking Insurance Into Account ................................................................ 24

CHAPTER TWO ................................................... 27

  SURGICAL METHODS FOR INTRAOPERATIVE PLACEMENT .................................................... 27

    Surgical Method For Implant Placement: Step-By-Step ..................................................................... 27

    Options For Anesthesia And Pain Control .......... 29

    Methods For Sinus Lifts And Bone Grafting ......... 30

    Guidelines For Post-Operative Care And Recovery ........................................................................... 33

CHAPTER THREE ................................................ 35

  RESTORATION AND PROSTHETIC OPTIONS ......... 35

   Kinds Of Prosthetics Supported By Implants ....... 35

   Material Selection For Prosthetics ...................... 36

   Fit And Personalization Of The Prosthetic ........... 37

   The Steps Involved In Securing The Prosthetic To The Implant .................................................... 38

   Upkeep And Handling Of Prosthetics Supported By Implants ........................................................ 40

## CHAPTER FOUR .................................................... 43

### SCIENTIFIC APPLICATIONS AND TECHNOLOGIES . 43

   Compact Dental Implants: Their Uses ................ 43

   Various Full-Arch Restoration Methods, Including All-On-4 .......................................................... 44

   Computer-Assisted Implant Procedures .............. 45

   Advances In Implant Surface Technology ........... 46

   Prospective Developments In Dental Implants .... 47

## CHAPTER FIVE ..................................................... 49

### MANAGING DENTAL IMPLANT SURGERY COMPLICATIONS AND FAILURES ........................ 49

   Typical Issues And Their Root Causes ................ 49

   Preventing And Identifying Issues Early ............. 50

   Options For Peri-Implantitis Treatment ............. 51

- Techniques For Removing And Replacing Implants ................................................................. 52
- Patient Instruction For Sustainable Outcomes ..... 53

## CHAPTER SIX .................................................................... 55

### AFTER SURGERY MANAGEMENT AND CARE .......... 55

- Instructions For Immediate Post-Operative Care . 55
- Extended-Term Dental Hygiene Procedures ........ 56
- Frequent Examinations And Expert Cleanings ..... 57
- Dietary Guidelines For Patients Receiving Implants ................................................................................ 58
- Identifying Indications Of Possible Problems ...... 59

## CHAPTER SEVEN ................................................................ 61

### CASE STUDIES AND PATIENT EXPERIENCES ........ 61

- Actual Patient Narratives And Results ................ 61
- Complex Implant Surgery Case Studies .............. 63
- Testimonies And Input From Those Who Have Received Implants ............................................. 64
- Dental Implants' Psychological And Social Effects ................................................................................ 66
- Images Of The Before And After And Visual Records ............................................................ 67

CHAPTER EIGHT .................................................... 71
  FAQS AND COMMON QUESTIONS ABOUT DENTAL
  IMPLANTS ........................................................... 71
    Pain Control And Recuperation Period ................. 71
    Durability And Extended Life Of Implants ........... 72
    Managing Dental Implants In The Course Of Daily
    Life ................................................................ 73
    Prices And Specifics Of Insurance Coverage ....... 74
    Dispelling Myths And False Ideas Regarding Dental
    Implants ......................................................... 75

## CONCERNING THIS BOOK

"Dental Implant Surgery" is a vital resource for contemporary dentists, providing a thorough understanding of implantology from its historical foundations to its most advanced technology. The book starts with a fascinating tour through the history of dental implants, outlining the significant innovations that have impacted the industry. It describes several kinds of implants, like endosteal and subperiosteal, and highlights the benefits and uses of each. The book emphasizes the importance of materials like titanium and zirconia, which are critical to guaranteeing the durability and success rates of implants.

Carefully considered diagnostic processes and treatment planning are covered, with a focus on the critical importance of first consultations and modern imaging methods such as CT and X-rays. The incorporation of digital planning tools emphasizes a customized treatment plan, which is reinforced by in-depth conversations about insurance and cost estimates, guaranteeing accessibility for a range of patient requirements.

The book's main focus is on surgical techniques for implant placement, which offer a thorough, step-by-step description of the processes. The guide navigates through complications, covering everything from anesthetic alternatives to sophisticated procedures like bone grafting and sinus lifts. It differentiates between implant placements that happen right away and those that happen later. It is backed by thorough post-operative care protocols that put the comfort and recuperation of the patient first.

The prosthetic alternatives and restoration section explores the artistry involved in creating dentures, bridges, and crowns supported by implants. To provide optimal functionality and aesthetics, it carefully addresses material selection, personalization, and the smooth integration of prosthetics with implants. The comprehensive maintenance regimens emphasize the significance of ongoing care in maintaining the best possible dental health.

The future of dental implantology is shown by developments in implant procedures and technologies, ranging from tiny implants to very advanced computer-guided surgeries. The book provides a forward-looking viewpoint that improves clinical practice and patient outcomes by examining advancements in implant surface technology and predicting new trends.

The text provides practitioners with crucial insights into the prevention, early detection, and efficient therapy of peri-implantitis by candidly addressing complications and failures. It highlights the critical role that educated patient care plays in reducing risks and improving treatment outcomes, emphasizing patient education as a cornerstone for guaranteeing long-term success.

Finally, "Dental Implant Surgery" integrates technical know-how with patient-centered care, making it a seminal work in the field of dental literature. Its thorough methodology, enhanced by case studies, real-world FAQs, and patient experiences, promotes a greater comprehension of the significant influence dental implants have on oral health and quality of life. This book is a valuable tool for dentists navigating the difficult field of implantology; it has the potential to improve patient outcomes and provide dentists more influence globally.

Overview of Dental Implants

Dental implants, which provide a long-lasting and aesthetically beautiful remedy for tooth loss, have completely transformed the profession of dentistry.

These surgical elements are made to fit into the jawbone and provide a strong base for different dental prostheses, like bridges, crowns, and dentures. To get the best possible integration and functionality, receiving a dental implant requires careful planning and execution. It can be easier to understand this sophisticated dental treatment if you are aware of the types, materials, success rates, history, and basic anatomy of dental implants.

Dental Implant Development and History

Dental implants have been around for thousands of years. The first attempts attempted inserting different materials into the jawbone; nevertheless, major progress was not achieved until the 20th century. Per-Ingvar Brånemark, a Swedish orthopedic surgeon, discovered in the 1950s that titanium could form a strong link with bone, a process known as osseointegration. This finding opened the door for contemporary dental implants, with the first one being successfully inserted in 1965. Since then, advancements in materials, methods, and success rates have led to a substantial evolution in dental implant technology, establishing it as a common alternative for tooth replacement.

An Overview of the Various Implant Types

Dental implants mostly come in two varieties: endosteal and subperiosteal.

The most prevalent kind of implants are endosteal ones, which are inserted straight into the mandible. Usually, they have the shape of screws, cylinders, or plates. Individuals with adequate bone density and height are good candidates for endosteal implants.

Subperiosteal Implants: These are implants that sit above the mandible but below the gingiva. They are made up of a metal framework that holds the prosthesis in place with posts that poke through the gums. Patients who are unable to undergo bone augmentation treatments or who have insufficient bone height can benefit from subperiosteal implants.

Frequently Used Materials for Implants

The materials chosen have a major impact on the longevity and success of dental implants. Zirconia and titanium are the materials most frequently utilized.

Titanium: The human body can tolerate this metal rather well since it is highly biocompatible. The exceptional osseointegration characteristics, strength, and longevity of titanium implants are well recognized. Because of their established track record of accomplishment, they have been the go-to option for decades.

Zirconia: A ceramic that provides an alternative to metal, zirconia is a more recent material in the dental implant industry. Additionally, it offers good osseointegration and is biocompatible. Because zirconia implants resemble natural teeth and are less likely to be visible through gum tissue, they are well-known for their aesthetic qualities. They also withstand heat and corrosion.

## Overall Success Rates and Implant Lifespan

Dental implants have a high success rate, usually in the range of 95% to 98%. These high success rates are a result of various factors, such as the

patient's oral health and dedication to post-surgery care, the dental surgeon's ability, and the quality of the materials utilized. Another important benefit of dental implants is their lengthy lifespan; given the right maintenance, they can last a lifetime. Implant integrity can be preserved with the help of routine dental exams, proper oral hygiene, and abstaining from bad habits like smoking.

## Fundamental Anatomy of a Device

Determining the fundamental structure of a dental implant can aid in simplifying the process. The fixture, abutment, and crown are the three basic components that make up a dental implant.

Fixture: This is the actual implant, a screw-shaped instrument that is surgically placed into the mandible. The fixture, which is made of zirconia or titanium, osseointegrates with the bone to act as the artificial tooth's root. This procedure, which usually takes many months, guarantees a solid base for the remainder of the implant.

Abutment: An abutment is affixed following the fixture's satisfactory integration with the mandible. The fixture is connected to the crown via the abutment, which acts as a connection. It offers a strong foundation for the crown by protruding over the gum line.

Crown: The dental implant's visible portion is made to resemble a real tooth in both appearance and functionality. The crown is crafted to match the patient's natural teeth in terms of color, shape, and size using materials like porcelain or ceramic, guaranteeing a seamless and aesthetically beautiful appearance.

Gaining knowledge about dental implant types, histories, compositions, rates of success, and anatomy can help you better understand this revolutionary dental treatment. Dental implants considerably improve oral health and general quality of life by providing a dependable and long-lasting remedy for tooth loss.

# CHAPTER ONE

## PROCEDURES FOR DIAGNOSIS AND TREATMENT PLANNING

### First Appointment And Evaluation Of The Patient

An initial consultation is an essential first step towards guaranteeing the success of dental implant surgery. Your dentist or oral surgeon will perform a thorough examination of your oral health during this session. To find out if you are a good candidate for dental implants, a thorough examination of your teeth, gums, and jawbone is required.

To find any underlying issues that can influence the surgery or healing process, your medical history will also be examined. Talking about your current drugs and any allergies you may have is part of this. Your dentist will inquire about your expectations for the implant process as well as your dental history, including any prior treatments.

Your dental practitioner will evaluate your lifestyle and preferences in addition to your physical health. For example, they will assess how well you maintain your dental health following surgery and how well you practice oral hygiene. This thorough evaluation aids in customizing the treatment program to your unique requirements and situation.

### Utilization Of Diagnostic Imaging (CT And X-Rays)

Sophisticated diagnostic imaging methods are essential for the planning of dental implant procedures. For accurate planning, thorough images of your jawbone and adjacent structures are provided using X-rays and CT scans.

X-rays provide a good picture of your teeth and jawbone's state and point out any places that should be taken seriously, such as infection or bone loss. However, a CT scan may be suggested in more complicated instances. A CT scan yields a three-dimensional image, which facilitates a more thorough evaluation of the sinus cavities, nerve routes, and bone structure.

With the use of these pictures, the precise location of implants can be found, guaranteeing that they are placed in the best possible places to support prosthetic teeth. These diagnostic methods increase the likelihood of a successful outcome by helping to identify and address potential issues before surgery.

## Software And Tools For Digital Planning

Digital planning tools and software are very beneficial for modern dental implant treatments. By precisely planning and simulating the surgery, these tools improve precision and predictability.

The dentist can make a virtual representation of your mouth with sophisticated software. The information gathered during your diagnostic imaging procedure is used to create this model.

The dentist can precisely plan each implant's location, angle, and depth thanks to the program. It also aids in helping you visualize the finished product, providing you with a clear expectation.

Surgical guidelines are made easier by digital planning tools and are utilized during the process to guarantee that the implants are positioned precisely as planned. These guidelines help ensure that there is less room for error and that the procedure goes well overall.

### Formulating A Personalized Therapy Program

Your dentist will develop a customized treatment plan after gathering and evaluating all the diagnostic data that is required. The steps in your dental implant surgery are described in this plan, which is made especially for your particular requirements and situation.

The quantity of implants needed, where they will be placed, and what kind of prosthetic teeth will be utilized will all be specified in the treatment plan. It will also cover any potential prerequisite operations, such as sinus surgery or bone grafting.

lift, to guarantee that there is enough bone to hold the implants.

The treatment plan will also outline the timetable for every step of the procedure, from the first operation to the last implantation of the prosthetic teeth.

Your dentist will walk you through each stage, outlining what to anticipate and how to get ready.

This all-inclusive strategy assists in controlling expectations and guarantees that you are well-informed about the process.

## Estimating Costs And Taking Insurance Into Account

Patients must comprehend the cost implications of dental implant surgery. Your dentist will provide you with a thorough cost estimate for the full operation during the treatment planning phase. This quote will cover the price of the implants as well as any necessary preoperative care and follow-up appointments.

It's crucial to talk about financing alternatives and payment schedules that might be available to lower the cost of the treatment. Payment plans that let you spread the cost across several months are offered by many dental offices.

Insurance policies can differ greatly when it comes to dental implants. Certain dental insurance policies might pay for some or all of the implants, particularly if they are considered medically necessary. However, other plans might not. Your dentist's office can help you through the claims process and confirm your insurance coverage. Additionally, they can offer proof and assistance for any required pre-authorizations.

You may plan and feel less stressed financially by being aware of the charges and your insurance coverage upfront. This will free you up to concentrate on your treatment and recovery.

Your dental implant surgery will be as successful and seamless as possible thanks to each of these processes in the diagnostic and treatment planning phases. Your dental team wants to provide you with a simple and quick route to a happier, healthier smile. To that end, they will evaluate your oral health in detail, make use of cutting-edge imaging and digital technologies, design a customized treatment plan, and give you a clear idea of how much treatment will cost.

# CHAPTER TWO

## SURGICAL METHODS FOR INTRAOPERATIVE PLACEMENT

### Surgical Method For Implant Placement: Step-By-Step

A thorough examination precedes the dental implant placement process. To evaluate the state of your jawbone and choose the ideal location for the implant, your dentist will conduct a comprehensive examination of your mouth, which may include obtaining X-rays and 3D scans.

Preparation: The dentist will make sure the region is sterile and clean before the procedure. To ensure you don't experience any pain throughout the treatment, a local anesthetic will be used to numb the surgical region.

Incision and Flap Elevation: To reveal the bone, the dentist will make a little incision in the gum tissue. After that, the gum tissue is delicately raised to form a flap that lets the jawbone show through.

Making the Pilot Hole Drill:

At the designated spot, a pilot hole is bored into the mandible. Extreme caution is used when performing this procedure to prevent harm to nearby structures including sinuses and nerves.

Increasing the Pilot Hole Size:

A sequence of drills is used to gradually expand the pilot hole. This produces an area big enough to fit the implant.

Implant Placement: The tiny titanium post that serves as the dental implant is inserted into the hole that has been made. Because titanium osseointegrates (integrate nicely with bone) well, it is used in many applications.

Suturing: The gum tissue is moved over the implant and sutured once the implant is in place. Usually, the stitches come out in seven to ten days.

Healing Period: It may require several months for osseointegration to occur. The implant solidifies into the jawbone throughout this period.

## Options For Anesthesia And Pain Control

Various forms of anesthesia can be used for dental implant surgery, depending on the patient's request and the intricacy of the operation.

The most popular kind of anesthesia for dental implant surgery is local anesthesia. It numbs the precise region of the mouth where the implant is going to be inserted so you may be awake and pain-free.

Sedation Anesthesia: Sedation anesthesia may be utilized for individuals who are experiencing anxiety or who are having a more involved operation.

This can be inhaled, intravenously, or orally delivered. As a result of the relaxation and partial consciousness it produces, you won't be cognizant of the process.

General Anesthesia: In rare circumstances, especially during lengthy surgical procedures, general anesthesia may be required. During the procedure, you are unconscious thanks to this technique.

After surgery, pain control is essential for a comfortable recovery. Often, over-the-counter medications like acetaminophen or ibuprofen are adequate.

Your dentist could occasionally recommend heavier painkillers. Applying ice packs to the outside of the face can aid in the reduction of soreness and edema.

## Methods For Sinus Lifts And Bone Grafting

Bone grafting is frequently needed when the jawbone is not strong enough to support an implant.

Bone Grafting: To strengthen the jaw's bone structure, bone material is added. The material used for the graft may be from a donor, another area of your body, or synthetic materials. This process aids in laying a strong basis for the implant.

Sinus Lifts: A sinus lift may be required for implants in the upper jaw, especially those near the molars and premolars.

This entails raising the sinus membrane and supplementing the sinus floor with bone graft material.

The amount of bone that is available to firmly anchor the implant is increased by this process.

Before the implant can be inserted, bone grafting and sinus lift both need more healing time—typically several months.

Implant Placement: Instant vs. Delayed

Implant insertion timing can change based on a person's unique situation.

Immediate Implant Placement: In this case, the implant is inserted right away following a tooth extraction. This method can shorten the duration of treatment and support bone preservation. On the other hand, it needs enough bone density and no infection.

Postponed Implant insertion:

With this method, the implant is placed after the extraction site has healed for a few months. When bone grafting is required or there is an infection, this is frequently required. It guarantees a more steady and dependable result.

# Guidelines For Post-Operative Care And Recovery

Sufficient aftercare is necessary for both a speedy healing process and the long-term viability of your dental implants.

Oral Hygiene: Use a soft toothbrush to gently brush the surgery site to maintain appropriate oral hygiene. For a few days, refrain from putting toothpaste directly on the area. To keep the region clean, rinse your mouth with an antibacterial mouthwash.

Diet: To prevent pressure on the surgery site, limit your intake to soft meals during the first few days. Reintroduce harder meals gradually as the healing process advances. Alcohol and hot drinks should be avoided as they may irritate the surgical site.

Refrain from Smoking: Smoking raises the risk of implant failure and can seriously hinder the healing process. It is very advised to abstain from smoking while recovering.

Follow-Up Appointments: Keep track of the healing process and make sure the implant is integrating well by attending all of your dentist's scheduled follow-up appointments.

You may guarantee the greatest potential outcome for your dental implants by adhering to these recommendations and scheduling routine dental examinations.

# CHAPTER THREE

## RESTORATION AND PROSTHETIC OPTIONS

### Kinds Of Prosthetics Supported By Implants

Patients considering dental implants have a variety of prosthetic choices to choose from, each designed to fulfill particular dental requirements. The three main categories of prostheses supported by implants are dentures, bridges, and crowns.

A single lost tooth is replaced with a crown. The crown, which is made to resemble the color and shape of your original teeth, is placed on top of the implant, which serves as the root. Patients who have one or more missing teeth dispersed across their mouths might consider this option.

Bridges can be used to replace several neighboring teeth. In a bridge, several strategically positioned implants support a succession of connected crowns.

When multiple teeth are lost in a row, this technique works very well to ensure a sturdy and durable replacement.

Patients who are missing most or all of their teeth can utilize dentures, either full or partial. Because implant-supported dentures are fixed to the implants, they are more sturdy and pleasant than standard dentures because they don't slip and offer superior comfort and function.

## Material Selection For Prosthetics

For dental prostheses, selecting the appropriate materials is essential for both functionality and aesthetics. The materials that are most frequently utilized include acrylic resin, zirconia, and porcelain.

Because of its robustness and organic appearance, porcelain is preferred. Being extremely durable and nearly resembling the translucency of actual teeth, it is a great material option for crowns and bridges.

Another well-liked choice is zirconia, which is renowned for its remarkable strength and biocompatibility. It's frequently utilized for bridges and crowns since it offers a strong solution that looks natural and can endure strong biting forces.

Usually, denture bases are made of acrylic resin. It can be dyed to resemble the color of natural gums and is lightweight, which improves the prosthesis' overall appearance.

## Fit And Personalization Of The Prosthetic

Implant-supported prosthetics must be fitted and customized in several ways to provide a precise fit and comfortable fit. First, the dentist measures and takes exact impressions of your mouth. These are employed to produce an intricate model that directs the prosthetics' design.

Precise customization is made possible by cutting-edge technologies like digital imaging and CAD/CAM

(Computer-Aided Design/Computer-Aided Manufacturing). These instruments guarantee that the prosthetics blend in perfectly with your real teeth and gums, giving them a natural look and maximum functionality.

The prosthetic is tried in your mouth during the fitting procedure to see whether any modifications are required. To guarantee comfort, good biting alignment, and aesthetics, this step is essential. All required adjustments are done before the last attachment.

## The Steps Involved In Securing The Prosthetic To The Implant

A crucial step in the dental implant process that calls for skill and accuracy is attaching the prosthesis to the implant. After the implant and jawbone have completely fused, a process termed osseointegration that usually takes many months, the operation starts.

An abutment is first placed on the implant in cases of crowns and bridges. This little connecting element acts as the prosthetic's foundation.

After that, dental cement or screws are used to firmly affix the crown or bridge to the abutment, guaranteeing a stable and long-lasting fit.

Dentures supported by implants are a little bit different. They frequently employ a ball or bar attachment mechanism.

A thin metal bar that fits over your jaw's curve and is fastened to the implants is called the bar attachment.

For stability, the denture clamps into this bar. Each implant includes a ball-shaped attachment called a ball attachment, which slides into matching sockets on the denture to guarantee a tight fit.

# Upkeep And Handling Of Prosthetics Supported By Implants

The durability of implant-supported prosthetics and your dental health depends on proper maintenance and care. Maintaining proper oral hygiene and scheduling routine dental exams are essential.

Daily brushing and flossing are essential to preventing gum disease and plaque buildup around crowns and bridges.

Effective cleaning around implants can be achieved with the use of specialized flossing instruments, such as water flossers or interdental brushes.

Dentures supported by implants need a little different maintenance. They do not require the same level of cleaning as regular dentures, but they still need to be taken out every night.

Food particles and plaque can be avoided by using a soft toothbrush to brush the dentures and clean the area surrounding the attachments.

Frequent dental checkups enable your dentist to verify the prosthetics and implants are still in good shape by examining their integrity. Your dentist can also maintain the health and operation of your dental implants by doing thorough cleanings and quickly taking care of any problems.

# CHAPTER FOUR

## SCIENTIFIC APPLICATIONS AND TECHNOLOGIES

### Compact Dental Implants: Their Uses

A notable development in the field of dental implantology is the use of mini dental implants or MDIs. These implants provide a less intrusive option for patients who might not have enough bone mass for regular implants because of their smaller diameter than typical implants.

To stabilize dentures and offer a more snug fit without the need for adhesives, small dental implants are commonly utilized. Additionally, they are perfect for confined areas where conventional implants cannot be positioned.

Mini dental implant insertion is typically a less intrusive process requiring only local anesthetic and a quicker recovery period. Many people find small dental implants to be a practical alternative since they can typically be placed in a single visit, requiring less bone than traditional implants. They offer a flexible option for a variety of dental restoration requirements and can also be utilized for single-tooth replacements in spaces with limited space.

## Various Full-Arch Restoration Methods, Including All-On-4

Using only four implants, the All-on-4 treatment is a novel full-arch restoration method that offers a whole set of teeth. To maximize contact with the bone and offer stable support for the prosthesis, this procedure strategically places two straight implants in the anterior region and two angled implants in the posterior region. Because this method eliminates the need for bone grafting, it is especially advantageous for patients who have experienced severe bone loss.

Additional full-arch restoration methods are the All-on-6 and All-on-8, which support the prosthesis with six or eight implants, respectively. These techniques provide more stability and might be chosen by patients with more demanding functional needs or those with particular anatomical needs. With the use of full-arch restoration procedures, a patient's confidence in their ability to eat, speak, and smile is increased.

## Computer-Assisted Implant Procedures

One important technical development in dental implantology is computer-guided implant surgery. Using cutting-edge imaging methods like cone beam computed tomography (CBCT), this method generates an accurate three-dimensional (3D) model of the patient's jaw.

With the use of this model, surgeons may precisely plan where to place implants, guaranteeing that the implants are positioned by the patient's bone structure and anatomical features.

To create a personalized surgical guide, a comprehensive digital scan of the patient's mouth is the first step in the procedure. By guiding the surgeon during the process, this aid improves accuracy and lowers the possibility of problems. By guaranteeing exact implant placement, lowering the possibility of nerve injury, and limiting the need for extensive bone grafting, computer-guided surgery improves results. Additionally, it expedites the length of the procedure and the recuperation period, giving patients a more effective and enjoyable experience.

## Advances In Implant Surface Technology

The integration of implants with bone tissue has been improved through the major evolution of implant surface technology. The surfaces of contemporary implants have undergone specific treatment to facilitate osseointegration—the process by which the implant integrates with the jawbone. Sandblasting, acid etching, and the use of bioactive coatings are examples of surface treatments that promote bone development and enhance stability.

One of the more recent developments is the creation of nanostructured surfaces, which improve cellular responses by imitating the environment of genuine bone. Osteoblasts, the cells that produce bones, are drawn to these surfaces, which speeds up the healing process and ensures stability over the long run. Furthermore, to lower the risk of infection and increase the success rates of dental implant treatments, some implants now have antibacterial coatings.

## Prospective Developments In Dental Implants

Technology and materials science will likely drive further breakthroughs in dental implantology in the future. The use of biomimetic materials, which aim to mimic the characteristics of natural bone and improve osseointegration, is one developing trend. To encourage bone repair and enhance implant stability, researchers are also looking into the possibilities of tissue engineering and stem cell therapy.

The application of artificial intelligence (AI) to digital dentistry is another exciting field. Artificial intelligence (AI) systems can evaluate patient data to forecast results and personalize treatment regimens, improving the accuracy and effectiveness of implant treatments. Furthermore, personalized implants and prosthetics are being made with 3D printing technology, providing a high level of customization and enhancing patient outcomes.

Dental implantology is expected to change as a result of these advancements, continuing research, and clinical trials. Procedures will become more successful, predictable, and minimally invasive. Patients should anticipate more sophisticated options for teeth restoration and quality of life enhancements as technology advances.

# CHAPTER FIVE

## MANAGING DENTAL IMPLANT SURGERY COMPLICATIONS AND FAILURES

### Typical Issues And Their Root Causes

Even though dental implant surgery is usually successful, problems can occasionally arise. Infection, implant failure, nerve injury, and sinus troubles are among the most frequent concerns. Poor oral hygiene following surgery or germs entering the incision during surgery can also result in infection at the implant site.

Inadequate bone support, incorrect implant placement, or high implant stress are common causes of implant failure. Implants positioned too near to nerves may, however rarely, cause nerve injury that results in numbness or pain. Implants in the upper jaw that protrude into the sinus cavity may cause sinus issues.

## Preventing And Identifying Issues Early

A comprehensive preoperative plan and patient evaluation are the first steps in preventing problems. Lowering the risk of infection during surgery can be achieved by ensuring the patient maintains good dental hygiene and is free of gum disease.

Employing sophisticated imaging methods, such as CT scans, aids in precisely arranging implant placement to prevent problems with the nerves and sinuses. Following surgery, patient education is essential. Patients should receive ongoing monitoring and instruction on good oral hygiene.

Vigilant observation for indications of infection, implant mobility, atypical pain, or changes in sensation is necessary for the early discovery of issues. By promptly attending to these indicators, minor problems can be avoided before they worsen.

## Options For Peri-Implantitis Treatment

An inflammatory disorder called peri-implantitis affects the hard and soft tissues around an implant, potentially resulting in implant failure and bone loss. It's imperative to intervene early. One of the available treatment options is mechanical debridement, which involves cleaning the implant surface of calculus and bacterial biofilm.

Antimicrobial treatments, including systemic antibiotics or antibiotic rinses, can aid in the management of infection. An additional method that offers accurate and least invasive decontamination is laser therapy.

In severe situations, bone loss may need to be replaced by surgically removing diseased tissue.

Following therapy, it's critical to continue practicing strict oral hygiene to avoid recurrence.

## Techniques For Removing And Replacing Implants

It may be required to remove and replace an implant if it fails. Using specialist equipment, the implant is unscrewed and extracted during the removal process so as not to harm the surrounding bone.

If there is bone deterioration, other treatments such as bone grafting would be needed to prepare the area for the implantation of future implants.

To enable the region to heal after the removal, a healing period is necessary. A replacement implant can be inserted if adequate bone growth and healing have occurred.

During this phase, precise planning and implementation guarantee a higher success rate for the replacement implant.

# Patient Instruction For Sustainable Outcomes

The key to long-term success is teaching patients about the upkeep and care of their dental implants. To avoid plaque accumulation and infection, patients should be made aware of the need to practice good oral hygiene, which includes brushing and flossing regularly.

They must be counseled against engaging in behaviors like smoking, teeth grinding, or chewing on tough foods that can put stress on the implant. To keep an eye on the condition of the implants and the tissues around them, routine dental examinations and expert cleanings are essential.

Teaching patients how to spot early warning indicators of problems, such as unusual discomfort or swelling, encourages timely referral to a professional, guaranteeing that any problems are dealt with efficiently.

# CHAPTER SIX

## AFTER SURGERY MANAGEMENT AND CARE

### Instructions For Immediate Post-Operative Care

The first 24 to 48 hours following dental implant surgery are critical for healing. It is normal for patients to have some discomfort and edema, but these can be controlled with prescription painkillers and applying cold packs to the affected area for 15 to 20 minutes at a time. To avoid difficulties, you must relax and refrain from excessive activity during this time.

Bleeding frequently occurs right after surgery. Until the bleeding stops, patients should gently bite on the gauze pads that their dentist has provided, changing them as needed. To reduce swelling, it's also a good idea to sleep with the head up. Steer clear of smoking, using straws, and spitting as these activities can disturb the blood clot and prevent it from healing.

It's important to maintain good oral hygiene. Maintaining the surgery site clean is facilitated by gently rinsing the mouth with a saline solution or an antiseptic mouthwash. To avoid irritating the surgery site, brushing should be done carefully. Observe any particular guidelines your dentist may have provided regarding using a particular toothbrush or rinse.

## Extended-Term Dental Hygiene Procedures

For dental implants to last a lifetime, good oral hygiene must be maintained. Patients should use fluoride toothpaste and a soft-bristled toothbrush to brush their teeth at least twice a day. To help ensure that no food particles or plaque accumulate, specialized interdental brushes or floss made for dental implants can be used to clean the area around the implant and the gum line.

Reducing germs and inflammation near the implant site can be achieved by regularly using an antimicrobial mouthwash. Maintaining the health of the surrounding tissues and implants also requires routine dental cleanings by a specialist. Your dental hygienist has to know about the implants to clean your teeth with the proper care.

## Frequent Examinations And Expert Cleanings

To keep an eye on the condition of dental implants, routine dental examinations are essential. Dentists generally advise seeing patients every six months, though specific situations may dictate a different schedule. The dentist will check the implants, surrounding gums, and general oral health during these appointments to make sure everything is in working order.

Expert cleanings hold similar significance. Dental hygienists are equipped with the knowledge and skills necessary to clean hard-to-reach areas with routine brushing and flossing. By eliminating tartar accumulation surrounding the implants, they can lower the chance of peri-implantitis, an infection that can result in implant failure.

## Dietary Guidelines For Patients Receiving Implants

An important factor in the healing process following dental implant surgery is diet. Patients should maintain a soft diet in the early postoperative days to prevent applying pressure to the surgery site. Smoothies, mashed potatoes, scrambled eggs, and yogurt are healthy choices. Steer clear of acidic, hot, or spicy foods since they may irritate the mending tissues.

Patients can progressively resume eating harder meals as their recuperation continues. But you must still refrain from eating anything too dense or sticky, as these can harm the implants or the surrounding bone.

The healing area can be better protected by chewing on the side of the mouth that is not the implant site.

## Identifying Indications Of Possible Problems

Understanding the warning indicators of possible complications might assist in guaranteeing timely care and avert more serious issues. Common warning indicators include bleeding that does not get better with time, edema, or chronic pain. Plus, redness, or soreness near the implant site could be signs of an infection.

You must notify your dentist right away if an implant feels loose or moves. A poor taste in the tongue, trouble eating, or changes in bite can also be signs of problems with the implants. Maintaining the health and longevity of your dental implants can be achieved by doing routine self-checks and promptly notifying your dentist of any unexpected symptoms.

# CHAPTER SEVEN

## CASE STUDIES AND PATIENT EXPERIENCES

### Actual Patient Narratives And Results

An invaluable source of information on the experience of having dental implant surgery is firsthand patient narratives.

These anecdotes frequently draw attention to the difficulties patients had before deciding to have implants, like trouble eating, self-consciousness about looks, or the inconvenience of having removable dentures.

Patients share how dental implants changed their lives and how they experienced this transformation.

One patient, Sarah, suffered for years due to a missing tooth, which impacted her self-esteem and her ability to chew food correctly.

She decided to have dental implants after speaking with her dentist and learning more about the process.

Sarah reported that the surgery was surprisingly painless, both during and after the procedure. Her smile and self-esteem were restored when she saw how natural her new tooth looked and felt.

John, a different patient, decided to get dental implants after having continuous problems with his dentures.

He dreaded having to take them off for cleaning because he felt uncomfortable wearing them. John talked about how much easier his daily life got following his implant procedure.

He felt more at ease in social situations and could indulge in his favorite meals without fear. In his testimony, he underlined how much dental implants had improved his quality of life.

## Complex Implant Surgery Case Studies

Case studies offer in-depth analyses of intricate dental implant procedures, demonstrating the skill of dental specialists and the creative methods employed to produce positive results. These studies frequently highlight difficult situations that require bone grafting to assure implant durability or numerous implants.

One noteworthy case study featured Mr. Smith, a patient who had suffered many tooth losses in an automobile accident.

In addition, there was damage to his jawbone, necessitating considerable restoration before the placement of implants.

The dental team used bone transplants to fill in the missing areas and highly modern imaging equipment to organize the procedure exactly.

Despite their intricacy, Mr. Smith's implants eventually merged seamlessly with his bone, regaining both appearance and functionality.

In a different case study, Mrs. Johnson sought out dental implants following years of discomfort and soreness from her regular dentures.

Her gum health and bone density have to be carefully taken into account. To guarantee the best outcomes, the dental team created a personalized treatment strategy that includes thoughtful prosthesis design and implant placement.

The favorable result for Mrs. Johnson demonstrated the value of careful planning and individualized treatment in implant dentistry.

## Testimonies And Input From Those Who Have Received Implants

Implant recipients' comments and testimonials offer insightful viewpoints on the complete patient experience, from the first consultation through the aftercare phase.

These testimonies frequently highlight things like pain control, recuperation duration, and contentment with the outcome. Good comments can reassure potential clients about the advantages of selecting dental implants.

Many patients thank implants for improving their ability to chew food and for their improved appearance. For example, Mr. Brown talked about how getting implants restored his confidence in his smile and how the process was unexpectedly easy and painless. His testimonies inspired others to think about getting implants to take the risk to improve their quality of life.

In a similar vein, Mrs. Lee emphasized the encouraging treatment she had from her dental team during the implant procedure. Their sympathetic approach and in-depth explanations helped her feel less anxious about having surgery. The favorable result for Mrs. Lee served as more evidence of the value of open communication and confidence between dental practitioners and patients.

## Dental Implants' Psychological And Social Effects

Dental implants have significant psychological and social effects that frequently improve patients' self-esteem and general well-being. Beyond the obvious advantages, such as better speech and chewing, implants can have a favorable impact on how people view themselves and relate to others.

Studies indicate that a considerable number of patients report a marked improvement in their self-esteem following the placement of dental implants. Having a smile that looks natural and feels safe and at ease is the source of this newly discovered confidence.

Patients frequently report feeling less self-conscious about their appearance and more at ease in social settings.

Furthermore, having dental implants might lessen the emotional strain of having to live with unpleasant dentures or missing teeth. Patients no longer have to be concerned about their teeth falling out or slipping, which can be embarrassing. People have a higher quality of life and are more inclined to fully participate in social activities and interpersonal relationships when they feel secure and free.

## Images Of The Before And After And Visual Records

Visual documentation and before-and-after pictures are essential for showcasing the revolutionary results of dental implants.

Prospective patients can see from these pictures what to anticipate in terms of both usefulness and aesthetics from the treatment.

Before and after pictures frequently show gaps in the grin or overt indications of tooth loss, which can affect the symmetry and structure of the face. Following dental implant placement, patients frequently have a smile that complements their facial features and seems natural.

The images demonstrate how the implants blend in perfectly with the neighboring teeth, improving the overall appearance of the face.

The procedure of implant implantation and the healing phases are also depicted visually, providing information about the recovery and prosthesis attachment timetable.

These pictures reassure patients about the treatment's predictability and assist them in visualizing the steps necessary to achieve their desired result.

Dental practitioners can effectively convey the advantages of implants and instill confidence in prospective patients who want to improve the appearance of their smile and oral health by providing thorough visual evidence.

# CHAPTER EIGHT

## FAQS AND COMMON QUESTIONS ABOUT DENTAL IMPLANTS

### Pain Control And Recuperation Period

Patients frequently worry about how they will manage their pain both during and after dental implant surgery. During the process, local anesthetic is usually administered to make sure you are comfortable and pain-free. Though there could be some pressure or vibrations, most discomfort is usually not very bad. It's common to have some stiffness and moderate swelling following the procedure; these can be treated with over-the-counter painkillers that your oral surgeon or dentist recommends.

Recovery times vary based on treatment complexity and personal recovery processes. After surgery, most people are usually able to resume their everyday activities and jobs a few days to a week later. To encourage healing and lower the chance of problems, it's critical to adhere to your dentist's recommendations for food, oral hygiene, and any recommended medications during the initial healing phase.

## Durability And Extended Life Of Implants

Dental implants are intended to be a permanent replacement for lost teeth. Implants can endure for decades or even a lifetime with the right maintenance and routine dental examinations. The implant is composed of biocompatible materials like titanium, which undergo a process known as osseointegration to fuse with the jawbone. Similar to a natural tooth root, its integration offers a sturdy basis.

Implant lifetime is also influenced by things like general health, lifestyle choices, and dental cleanliness routines. It is essential to practice proper oral hygiene, which includes seeing your dentist for professional cleanings and brushing and flossing regularly, to avoid issues like gum disease that can shorten the life of implants.

## Managing Dental Implants In The Course Of Daily Life

One advantage of dental implants is that they feel and work like real teeth, so you can smile, chew, and speak with assurance.

You can take care of the implant just like you would a natural tooth once it has completely healed and the final treatment (like a crown or bridge) has been placed. There are no dietary limitations, although it is advised to stay away from foods that are very hard or habits like biting ice that can harm the repair.

Keeping your teeth clean is crucial to the longevity of your implants. Plaque buildup can be avoided and the surrounding gums maintained by regularly brushing, flossing, and using antimicrobial mouthwash in the area around the implant and restoration.

## Prices And Specifics Of Insurance Coverage

The number of implants required, the difficulty of the process, and your geographic location are some of the variables that can affect the cost of dental implants. The surgical implantation of the implant, the abutment (connection) that joins the implant to the restoration, and the actual final restoration (like a crown or bridge) are usually involved.

Because of their longevity and natural appearance, dental implants are frequently a beneficial investment, even though they may first seem more expensive than other tooth replacement choices. Implants are generally covered in part by dental insurance plans, particularly if they are deemed medically necessary. It's crucial to speak with your insurance company to find out what is and isn't covered as well as potential out-of-pocket costs.

## Dispelling Myths And False Ideas Regarding Dental Implants

There are several false beliefs and misconceptions regarding dental implants that may cause patients to hesitate or have unwarranted fears. The idea that dental implants hurt is often spread. In actuality, local anesthetic ensures minimal discomfort during the treatment, and medication can efficiently manage any pain experienced afterward.

The idea that dental implants are inappropriate for elderly people is another common misunderstanding. As long as the candidate is in good general health and has sufficient jaw bone density, age is not a barrier to candidacy. Dental implants can restore dental function and improve the quality of life for older persons, just as they do for younger patients.

Dispelling the myth that dental implants need a lot of upkeep is also crucial. Implants do not deteriorate like natural teeth do, but they still require routine dental hygiene maintenance. Implants can offer a reliable and long-lasting replacement for lost teeth with the right upkeep.

Making educated decisions regarding your oral health can be facilitated by knowing about dental implants. Speaking with a skilled oral surgeon or dentist can help you receive advice and information that is particular to your requirements and concerns.

www.ingramcontent.com/pod-product-compliance
Lightning Source LLC
Chambersburg PA
CBHW071841210526
45479CB00001B/242